Metabolic Confusion Diet

The Easy Beginners Guide to Increasing Metabolic Rate for Weight Loss Including a 7-Day Meal Plan and Mouth-Watering Healthy Recipes

Ben Smith

Table of Contents

Disclaimer iv

Introduction 1

What are Metabolic Confusion Diets? 2

How Do Metabolic Confusion Diets Function? 4

Are Metabolic Confusion Diets Safe? 4

Advantages of Metabolic Confusion Diets 5

Seven Days Calorie (Cal) Confusion Meal Regimen 7

Recipes 24

    Massaged Kale Chickpea and Butternut Squash Pasta Salad 24

    Chicken Farro Salad 26

    BBQ Lentil Burgers and Ranch Dressing 28

    Fried Sage and Butternut Squash with Browned-Butter Gnocchi 30

    Peppers and Meatballs 32

    Buffalo Chicken Sandwich 34

    Bison Meatballs in Spicy Tomato Sauce 36

Blackened Salmon 38

Crockpot Chipotle Chicken Soup 41

Asparagus Tarts and Grill Crispy Lobster 43

Grilled Honey Lime Shrimp 46

Spicy Asian Zucchini with Noodles 48

Homemade Salmon Tacos and Salsa 50

Noodle Bowl with Keto Asian Barbecue Meatballs 54

Grilled Chicken Breasts with a Five-Ingredient Lemon Yogurt-Marinated 57

Oat Cakes with Turmeric Salmon 59

Sriracha Honey Dressing with Salad of Asian Beef 61

Foil Packets with Italian Chicken and Veggies 63

Steak Soup with Salsa Verde 66

Spicy Drunken Noodles 70

Banana Berry Breakfast Oat Bars 72

Feta Turkey Burgers with Caramelized Onion Spinach 76

Snapper a la Veracruz 79

Bear-Sized PB and J 81

Five Mins Spicy Tuna Rolls 82

Easy and Quick Turkey Noodle Soup 83

Cauliflower Enchiladas (Roasted) 85

Sea Salt and Lime Spinach Chips 87

Four-ingredient Veggies Egg Muffins 89

Sheet Pan Curried Chicken and Vegetables ... 90

Very Cherry Protein Shake 92

Chickpea, Butternut Squash, and Lentil Moroccan Stew 93

Low-carb Turkey Cabbage Rolls 95

Oven-roasted Butternut Squash 98

Strawberry Avocado Farro Salad 100

Golden Milk Chia Pudding 102

Perfect Steak Fajitas 103

Disclaimer

Please note that the information in this book are written for the express purpose of sharing educational information only. The information herein is based on research and stated to be reliable and consistent, but the author neither implies nor intends any guarantee of accuracy for specific cases or individuals.

It is recommended that you consult a licensed professional before beginning any practice relating to your health, diet, or lifestyle. The contents of this book are not replacement for professional advice.

The author, publisher and distributors disclaim any liability, loss or damage and risk taken by individuals who directly or indirectly act on the information contained in this book.

Introduction

One of the most recent fad dietary plans to gain traction on social networking sites is the "metabolic confusion" program. Like several other fad diets, it claims that you can shed some weight while consuming everything you'd like. Diet supporters argue that by alternating between high Cal (calorie) and low Cal days, you may also shed some weight while also boosting your body's metabolic reactions.

Metabolic confusion diets are comparable to intermittent fasting, except that they're without severe calorie restrictions. A dieter may, for instance, consume only 1200 Cal one day and 2,000 Cal the next. While there has not been sufficient study on the subject of metabolic confusion diets, we can link it to a common kind of intermittent fasting called the 5:2 diet, which involves eating normally for 5 days and then staying off food for 2 days or eating roughly five hundred Cal.

Irrespective of the fact that "feed periods" allow you to consume as much food as you want, folks might not feel any more famished and probably consume less total and less food on feed periods than they did prior to when they started intermittent fasting. This backs up the assumption that this type of fasting can help you lose weight in the same way that calorie-restricted daily diets do.

What are Metabolic Confusion Diets?

Metabolic confusion diets also called calorie cycling or calorie shifting, are based on switching lower and higher calorie consumption. They are based on the idea that you can fool your system into not slowing your metabolism and not boosting appetite.

The concept is that by altering the number of Cal your system processes, you'll help make your metabolism up-to-par with executing and boosting your basal metabolic rate (BMR), or the number of Cal your system consumes while you are resting. As a result, you'll be able to burn additional calories and lose weight.

A broad-licensed practitioner and a prominent author, Dr. Joel Furhman is a globally known authority on natural and nutrition health, tells Woman's Day that as soon as you achieve your optimal weight, your system will oppose shedding of weight. "This is accomplished by lowering your metabolism, thyroid, respiratory quotient, and body temperature."

How Do Metabolic Confusion Diets Function?

Metabolic confusion diets do not have any hard and fast guidelines. In 2 weeks, for instance, you may undertake eleven days of dedicated lower Cal consumption and then three days of greater Cal consumption. You may also conduct a 3-week low Cal followed by a 1-week high Cal cycle over the course of thirty days. There are no hard and fast rules about what foods to consume while utilizing the diet.

Are Metabolic Confusion Diets Safe?

If you're not suffering from any chronic health conditions, these diets are safe for you to attempt. Nevertheless, you need to always require medical advice before embarking on a fresh eating plan to ensure you are receiving the right calorific value for your weight and height.

"If you choose to adopt a new regimen, you need do so under the guidance of a physician, preferably a nutritionist who can ensure that you're obtaining enough nutrients." The number of Cal you need depends on your height and weight. For instance, if you are 6'5" and you are consuming 1,200 Cal on low Cal periods, you are practically starving yourself."

Advantages of Metabolic Confusion Diets

The benefits of the diet include the possibility that individuals who attempt metabolic confusion will keep practicing it for a lengthier period and become more fulfilled than individuals who just decrease Cal. But, there's no evidence that our metabolism may be confused. However, other people think that those few days when they can consume more prove to be vital for them.

One research assessed Cal shifting to Cal restriction and discovered that respondents consumed fewer Cal (forty-five percent fewer Cal in the Cal shifting group, fifty-five percent fewer Cal in the Cal restriction group), irrespective of whether they were attempting to "shift" instead of "**decrease**" their Cals. For 3 days in every fourteen days, the Cal shifting set did eat the amount of food as they liked, whereas the calorie restriction set did eat the very same Cal value daily. Although both subjects set to shed weight, the Cal shifting subject set felt less famished and more pleased than the Cal restriction group, according to the research. Furthermore, only fifteen percent of the Cal shifting group quit before the research was finished, compared to thirty-six percent of the Cal-restricted group.

Seven Days Calorie (Cal) Confusion Meal Regimen

Switch between high Cal periods with desserts containing two thousand Cals and low-calorie times with four meals of 1200-calories. When you eat more Cal, you get extra nutrients and minerals into your cellular structures, which helps you create muscle and speed up your metabolic rate. You reduce your Cal intake the following day, thereby transforming your system into a fat-shedding engine.

SUNDAY: High-Cal day (2000 Cal)

Breakfast

- One mid-sized orange (62 Cal)
- 1/4 cup of shredded cheddar cheese (low-fat) (49 Cal)

- One large-sized egg omelet (96 Cal)
- Two slices of turkey bacon (nitrite/nitrate-free) (70 Cal)
- One slice of whole-wheat bread (toasted) (100 Cal)

Total Calorific Value: (377 Cal)

Snack

- One tablespoon of peanut butter (95 Cal)
- 1.5 of larger rectangular graham crackers (three squares) (90 Cal)

Lunch

- One cup of baby carrots (50 Cal)
- Two slices of turkey-breast meat (44 Cal)
- Lettuce(5 Cal)
- One slice of American cheese(low-fat) (38 Cal)
- Two slices of whole-wheat bread (200 Cal)

- Two slices of tomato (6 Cal)
- One mid-sized banana (105 Cal)
- Four squares of dark chocolate, 70-85percent cocoa (72 Cal)

Snack

- Fifteen almonds (105 Cal)
- One mid-sized apple (95 Cal)

Dinner

- One cup of tomato sauce (78 Cal)
- ½ cup of broccoli (steamed) (27 Cal)
- Four oz. chicken breast (cooked) (186 Cal)
- ½ cup of zucchini (chopped) (10 Cal)
- One cup of whole-wheat spaghetti (cooked) (176 Cal)

Dessert

- Ten raspberries (10 Cal)
- One cup of frozen yogurt (low-fat) (280 Cal)

Total Calorific Value: 2,049

MONDAY: Low-Cal day (1200 Cal)

Breakfast

- One teaspoon of honey (usually 20 Cal)
- Raspberries (21 Cal)
- Single -yield reduced-fat Greek yogurt (plain) (150 Cal)
- Fifteen almonds (90 Cal)

Snack

- Five pita chips (65 Cal)
- Two tablespoons of hummus (50 Cal)

- Ten baby carrots (40 Cal)

Lunch

- Two rings of green bell peppers (4 Cal)
- One oz. OF part-skim mozzarella cheese (71 Cal)
- English Muffins (134 Cal)
- ¼ cup of pizza sauce (34 Cal)

Snack

- One tablespoon of peanut butter (usually 95 Cal)
- Little banana (90 Cal)

Dinner

- One tablespoon of teriyaki sauce (20 Cal)
- Three oz. salmon (121 Cal)
- ¼ cup of (uncooked) brown rice (172 Cal)

- ½ cup of broccoli (30 Cal)

Total Calorific Value: 1207

TUESDAY: High- Cal Day (2000 Cal)

Breakfast

- One tablespoon of strawberry jam (40 Cal)
- Two scrambled eggs plus ½ cup of asparagus (13 + 142 = 155 Cal)
- One slice of whole-wheat bread (100 Cal)
- ½ cup of blackberries (31 Cal)

Snack

- one honey graham cracker (59 Cal)
- one teaspoon of cinnamon plus pear slices (6 +103 = 109 Cal)

Lunch

Cal Zone

- Usually two oz. pizza dough (frozen) (160 Cal)
- One tablespoon of Rosemary (10 Cal)
- ¼ cup of ricotta cheese (part-skim) (85 Cal)
- ½ cup of spinach (steamed)(20 Cal)
- ½ cup of chicken breast (chopped) (138 Cal)
- One tablespoon of pizza sauce (9 Cal)

Snack

- One teaspoon of honey plus ½ cup of vanilla yogurt (low-fat) (21+ 104 = 125 Cal)
- One oz. cashews (150 Cal)

Dinner

- One oz. whole wheat roll (74 Cal)
- Three oz. of lean beef (120 Cal)

- One cup of lima beans (176 Cal)
- ½ cup of potatoes plus one teaspoon of dill, one tablespoon of parmesan cheese, as well as a pinch of salt (22 + 68 + 6 = 96 Cal)

Dessert

- One tablespoon of Nutella (95 Cal)

Total Calorific Value: 1962

WEDNESDAY: Low-Cal Day (1200 Cal)

Breakfast

- ½ cup of blueberries (42 Cal)
- Two organic waffles (frozen) (200 Cal)
- One tablespoon of maple syrup (50 Cal)

Snack

- Six slices of celery stick (6 Cal)

- One tablespoon of peanut butter (natural) (95 Cal)

- Twenty-five raisins (39 Cal)

Lunch

- Ten baby carrots (40 Cal)

- One cup of reduced-sodium contained in the tomato soup (158 Cal)

- One basil plus, one slice of Swiss cheese, and also a small whole-wheat pita(toasted) (1 +74 +106= 181 Cal)

Snack

- One mid-sized nectarine (62 Cal)

Dinner

- One tablespoon of hoisin sauce (35 Cal)
- Three oz. shrimp (90 Cal)
- ¼ cup of red peppers (12 Cal)
- ¼ cup of couscous (preferable to use uncooked than cooked) (163 Cal)
- ½ cup of peas (58 Cal)

Total Calorific Value: 1231 Cal

THURSDAY: High- Cal Day (2000 Cal)

Breakfast

- ¼ cup of mushrooms with ½ cup of sautéed potatoes (one tablespoon of olive oil) and one teaspoon of garlic powder and finally a dash of salt (119 + 58+ 9+ 4 = 190 Cal)
- One cup of orange juice (112 Cal)

- One slice of Canadian bacon (nitrite/nitrate-free) with a poached egg on a whole-wheat English muffin (43+71 +134 = 248 Cal)

Snack

- one tablespoon of almond butter with ½ wheat bagel (33 +150 = 183 Cal)
- Twenty-five raspberries (25 Cal)

Lunch

- One tablespoon of hummus (25 Cal)
- Whole-wheat wrap (190 Cal)
- Four olives (20 Cal)
- ½ cup of carrots (shredded) (25 Cal)
- ¼ cup of sprouts (2 Cal)
- Two oz. deli chicken breast (50 Cal)
- One clementine (35 Cal)

- ½ cup of romaine lettuce (shredded) (4 Cal)
- ¼ cup of pear (59 Cal)
- Eight cherries (40 Cal)

Snack

- One mozzarella cheese stick (part-skim) (70 Cal)
- ½ cup of edamame (65 Cal)

Dinner

- Three oz. baked trout plus lemon as well as ¼ cup of bread crumbs: (30 +126 = 156 Cal)
- ½ cup of kale (steamed) plus ¼ cup of brown rice as well as ¼ cup of chickpeas: (16 + 172 + 72 = 260 Cal)
- ½ cup of tomatoes (roasted) (22 Cal)

Dessert

- ½ cup of mango sherbet (120 Cal)
- One tablespoon coconut (shredded) (90 Cal)

Total Calorific Value: 1991 Cal

FRIDAY: Low- Cal Day (1200 Cal)

Breakfast

- Cinnamon oatmeal (170 Cal)
- Two large strawberries (sliced) (12 Cal)

Snack

- ½ cup of pumpkin seeds (roasted) (142 Cal)

Lunch

- Fourteen walnuts (halves) (185 Cal)
- One oz. feta cheese (58 Cal)
- ½ cup of broccoli (15 Cal)

- 1/3 cup of dried cranberries (sweetened) (138 Cal)
- One cup of spinach (7 Cal)
- One tablespoon of balsamic vinaigrette (light) (30 Cal)

Snack

- One tablespoon of peanut butter (95 Cal)
- Ten whole wheat crackers (90 Cal)

Dinner

- One cup of sweet potato (114 Cal)
- ½ chicken breast (grilled)(130 Cal)
- One cup of cauliflower (steamed) (25 Cal)

Total Calorific Value: 1221 Cal

SATURDAY: High- Cal Day (2000 Cal)

Breakfast

- One wedge honeydew melon (45 Cal)
- one oz. cheddar cheese plus two-egg omelet, two turkey sausage links (nitrite/nitrate-free), as well as ¼ cup of red peppers (chopped): (113 +142 + 132+ 6 = 387 Cal)
- One slice of whole-wheat toast plus one tablespoon raspberry preserves: (50 + 100 = 150 Cal)

Snack

- One cup of cinnamon wheat (shredded) (200 Cal)
- ½ cup of milk (low fat)(52 Cal)

Lunch

- Three oz. sliced chicken breast (grilled) (140 Cal)
- One cup of whole-wheat pasta (176 Cal)
- ½ cup of zucchini(10 Cal)

- ½ cup of marinara sauce (111 Cal)

Snack

- Fifty pistachios (160 Cal)

Dinner

- six artichoke hearts and ¼ cup of tomatoes (sundried) plus 1/3 cup of uncooked quinoa (20 + 160+ 35= 215 Cal)
- Whole wheat bun (120 Cal)
- Black bean veggie burger (115 Cal)
- Romaine leaf (1 Cal)
- Tomato slice (3 Cal)
- Onion ring (2 Cal)

Dessert

- Sixteen animal crackers (120 Cal)

- Prepared hot chocolate, made with water: (113 Cal)

Total Calorific Value: 2013 Cal

Recipes

Massaged Kale Chickpea and Butternut Squash Pasta Salad

Yield: 8

Ingredients

Massaged Kale Preparation

- 1 juiced lemon
- 1 bunch of chopped kale
- 1 tablespoon of lemon rosemary seasoning
- 1 tablespoon of olive oil (or lemon grapeseed oil)

Salad Preparation

- 1 tablespoon of olive oil
- 2 cups of already cut butternut squash
- 1 whole wheat pasta, set to package guidelines
- 1 tablespoon of lemon rosemary seasoning

- ¼ cup of pepita seeds

- 1/3 cup of dried cranberries

- 2 tablespoons of hemp seeds

- 2 tablespoons of divided lemon rosemary seasoning

- ¼ cup of olive oil or lemon grapeseed oil

Procedure

1. In a large dish, combine one tablespoon of lemon rosemary spice, lemon juice, one tablespoon of lemon olive oil, and the kale. Massage the kale leaves with your hands to incorporate the seasonings, lemon juice, and oil. Seal the dish with plastic wrapping material and chill for at least one hour after the leaves have been massaged well.

2. Put butternut squash chunks onto a sheet pan coated with nonstick wrap. Distribute the squash inside a uniform layer onto the pan, coated with olive oil and lemon rosemary spice. Preheat the

oven to 425 degrees Fahrenheit and bake the squash for thirty to thirty-five minutes, or until soft.

3. Prepare spaghetti while the squash roasts. To end the process of preparation, place the pasta over cold water after it has been drained.

4. Inside a large mixing basin, mix the squash, pasta, as well as additional ingredients. In a large mixing bowl, combine the kale you massaged earlier with the rest of the ingredients. Refrigerate for future use or eat right now.

Chicken Farro Salad

Yield: 4

Ingredients

- ½ cup of sesame dressing, bottled

- 8 ounces or 3 pouches of brown rice, quinoa, or microwavable farro

- 1 cup of small-diced cucumber, seedless

- 1 cup of green seedless grapes halved

- 2 tablespoons of fresh dill, chopped

- ¼ cup of flat-leaf parsley, chopped and fresh

- 1 pound of skinless boneless chicken breast strips, grilled

Procedure

1. Toss together the grapes, dressing, grain, dill, parsley, and cucumber in four storage units.
2. Sprinkle with pepper and salt to taste. Add the chicken on top. You can serve to hot at normal temperature or a low temperature. Preserve inside a closed container inside the refrigerator for about seven days and when you like.

BBQ Lentil Burgers and Ranch Dressing

Yield: 8 burgers

Ingredients

- 3 cloves of minced garlic
- 1/3 cup of white onion, chopped
- 2 teaspoons of dried parsley
- ¼ cup of tomato paste
- ¼ cup of BBQ sauce
- ½ cup of brown rice, cooked
- 1 ½ cup of GF breadcrumbs or whole-grain panko
- 1 large egg
- 10-12 divided whole wheat buns
- Onion, lettuce tomato (optional toppings)
- ¼ cup of ranch dip

Procedure

1. Toss lentils and garlic cloves, diced white onion, parsley, and tomato paste inside a large mixing basin. Toss everything together well.
2. Combine the big egg, BBQ sauce, and cooked brown rice inside a mixing bowl. Mix it up some more.
3. Fold in panko bread crumbs (3/4 cup) lightly. Put the rest of the bread crumbs inside a small dish to save for later.
4. Set aside and prepare two oven sheets with baking parchment after everything is incorporated.
5. Using a two-ounce scoop, divide the lentil combination into patties, carefully pressing every side into the residual panko breadcrumbs to produce a crunchy texture on the outside.
6. Place each of the patties onto the baking paper two inches apart and place in the fridge for one hour or up to 24 hours, covered.

7. Preheat your oven to 400°F when prepared to cook.

8. While your oven preheats, take out your baking papers from your refrigerator.

9. Place in the oven for twenty minutes, then remove, turn, and bake for another ten minutes, or till panko has lightened in color. Remove from the oven, chill for five minutes, and serve with your preferred whole grain bread and your preferred toppings!

Fried Sage and Butternut Squash with Browned-Butter Gnocchi

Yield: 2

Ingredients

- 2 fresh sage stems leaves

- ½ cup of canola oil

- 2 tablespoons of butter

- 1 pound of gnocchi

- 2 tablespoons of good-quality Parmesan, freshly grated

- 2 cups or 1 pound of chopped, peeled butternut squash

Procedure

1. Preheat the oil inside a small nonstick skillet over moderate-to-high heat. When it begins to shimmer, incorporate the sage and cook for one to two minutes, or until it becomes crispy. Move the sage leaves into a dish coated with paper towels for draining with a large spoon.
2. Heat the gnocchi as per package instructions inside a big nonstick pan of simmering salted water. Drain with care.

3. Melt the butter inside the same pan on moderate heat. Cook, turning the pan regularly, for two to three minutes, or until the buttery material is somewhat colored and smells like nuts. Cook, stirring occasionally until the squash is colored and fork-tender, approximately five minutes.
4. Bring back the gnocchi into the pan and thoroughly mix them up. Serve in dishes with Parmesan cheese and fried sage on top.

Peppers and Meatballs

Yield: 4

Ingredients

- ½ sliced onion

- 1 tablespoon of olive oil

- 1 sliced green pepper

- 1 sliced red pepper

- 1 tablespoon of Italian seasoning

- 3 cloves of minced garlic

- 1 pound of cooked Italian-style meatballs (such as Aidells or Al Fresco)

- 15 ounces or 2 tablespoons of a can of diced tomatoes or tomato paste

Procedure

1. Heat the oil in a large pan over medium-high heat until it shimmers. Garlic, peppers, onion, a few grinds of pepper, a huge pinch of salt, and Italian seasoning are added to the pan. Cook, turning occasionally, for approximately five minutes, or till the onions become transparent and the peppers become tender.

2. Add the tomato puree and heat for three minutes, or until it blackens. Add the tomatoes and half a

cup of water to the mixture and carefully nestle in the meatballs. Cook, covered, for about ten minutes, or until the meatballs are well cooked.

3. Divide the mixture into four containers and serve with a piece of bread.

Buffalo Chicken Sandwich

Yield: 1

Ingredients

- ½ cup of Greek yogurt

- ¼ cup of crumbled blue cheese

- Pepper and salt to taste

- Juice of half a lemon

- 1/2 tablespoon of chili powder

- 4 skinless, boneless chicken breasts (4 to 6 ounces each)

- 2 tablespoons of butter, melted in the oven for twenty seconds

- 1 sliced red onion

- 2 tablespoons of hot sauce

- 4 toasted sesame buns

- 4 lettuce leaves, romaine

Procedure

1. Preheat a grill pan or nonstick grill. Mix the lemon juice, yogurt, and blue cheese, as well as a sprinkle of pepper and salt, while the oven is cooking. Cast aside after stirring.
2. Sprinkle the breasts with salt, pepper, and chili powder. Cook for five to six minutes on one side before turning the chicken breasts over the heated grill.
3. Arrange the onion along the border of the grill. (If you are utilizing a grill pan, delay until the chicken

is removed before searing the onions.) Cook for another four to eight minutes, or until the chicken breast is solid and the fried onions are springy for touch. Place it on a platter with the onions you grilled.

4. Toss the butter and spicy sauce together and spread it everywhere on the chicken breast. Put inside a romaine leaf at the bottom of each bun. Add your chicken breast and a dollop of blue cheese sauce atop. Put the upper half of the sandwich and the fried onions.

Bison Meatballs in Spicy Tomato Sauce

Yield: 5

Ingredients

- ¼ minced onion

- 2 pounds of ground bison

- 2 cloves of minced garlic

- ¼ cup of Italian bread crumbs

- 1 egg

- ¼ cup of parsley, minced

- ½ cup of grated Parmesan

- 1 tablespoon of olive oil

- ¼ cup of basil, minced

- 1 sprig

- ¼ cup of red grape juice

- 28 ounces or 2 cans of whole tomatoes, hand-crushed

- 1 teaspoon of crushed red pepper flakes

Procedure

1. Toss together the first eight components in a mixing dish with three large pinches of pepper and

salt each. Combine and form into golf-ball-sized spheres using your hands. Refrigerate for thirty minutes before serving.

2. Heat oil in a saucepan over moderate-high heat. Put as much as you need. Sear both sides for roughly fifteen minutes, depending on how many meatballs could fit inside a layer. (If required, work in bunches.) Move to a paper towel-lined plate.

3. Pour the grape juice into the saucepan, scraping off any browned pieces with a wooden spatula. Reduce the temperature to a moderate low setting. Transfer the meatballs, as well as the basil sprig, red pepper flakes, and tomatoes, to the saucepan. Add the sauce and cook for thirty minutes with the cover on the pot. Serve with a side of sauce.

Blackened Salmon

Yield: 4

Ingredients

- 1 teaspoon of cumin

- 1 teaspoon of paprika

- 1 teaspoon of garlic powder

- 1 teaspoon of dark brown sugar

- ½ teaspoon of kosher salt

- ½ teaspoon of onion powder

- ¼ teaspoon of black pepper

- ¼ teaspoon of chili powder

- 1 tablespoon of olive oil

- 1 ½ pound skin-removed salmon fillet

- 1 teaspoon of chopped parsley

- 1 lime, sliced into 4 pieces

Procedure

1. Mix brown sugar, cumin, paprika, salt, onion powder, garlic powder, black pepper, and chili powder inside a small mixing dish.
2. Slice salmon fillets into four equal portions, each weighing around six ounces.
3. Sprinkle one teaspoon of the fille darkening seasoning mixture on every fillet side, for a total of two tsp.
4. Preheat big stainless steel or cast-iron pan over moderate-high heat. When the pan is heated, pour in the oil.
5. Put the fish fillets inside your pan and heat for two to three minutes, or until slightly browned and crispy.
6. Toss and heat for another one to two minutes, or until the Hesh easily flakes.
7. Move to a platter and garnish with parsley and a slice of lime.

Crockpot Chipotle Chicken Soup

Yield: 6

Ingredients

- ½ chopped medium onion

- 4 large chicken breasts (skinless, boneless)

- 15 fluid ounce 1 or can of drained black beans

- 3 sticks of small chopped celery

- 28 fluid ounces or 1 can of diced tomatoes plus juices

- 12 fluid ounces or 1 can of drained corn

- 2 chopped chipotle chilis + 1 tablespoon of adobo sauce

- 3 cloves of minced garlic

- Vegetable broth or 4 cups of chicken

- 1 teaspoon of chili powder

- Pepper and salt to taste

Serving/Garnish Suggestions

- Lime wedges (optional)

- 1 tablespoon of chopped cilantro

- Greek yogurt or Sour cream optional, to taste.

- Tortilla strips to taste (optional)

Procedure

1. Inside your slow cooker, combine all ingredients except the garnish ingredients. We suggest putting the chicken last to allow you thoroughly mix the broth before putting it.

2. Heat the soup for three to four hours on high heat or six to eight hours on low heat.

3. Remove the chicken from the slow cooker and divide it with two forks. Return it to your slow cooker. Cut the cilantro and toss it in with the other ingredients. As required, season the soup with

pepper and salt. Serve right away. We like to add a drop of lime juice to our, but it's not required. Soup can be frozen for up to three months.

Asparagus Tarts and Grill Crispy Lobster

Yield: 4

Ingredients

- ¼ pound of trimmed asparagus
- 1¼ pound of live lobster
- Flour
- 1/3 pound of fresh dough, available at a local pizza shop or grocery
- 1½ cup of fontina cheese, grated
- 1 cup of crème Fraiche
- Red pepper flakes, crushed
- 1 lemon

- Olive oil

- Dill

Procedure

1. Fill a big saucepan halfway with water and bring to a boil on high heat. When the water boils, add the lobster and simmer for eight minutes, or until the shells are brilliant red. Take the lobster out of the water and set it aside to cool before removing the flesh. Reserve the meat, which has been divided into easy-to-chew pieces.

2. Fill a moderately-sized saucepan halfway with water and bring to a boil. Put the asparagus inside the water and simmer for one minute, or until just soft. Take the asparagus out of the saucepan and shock it in cold water right away. Remove from the equation.

3. Heat the gas grill to moderate-low, direct heat, or, if using a charcoal grill, to the point where you can

place your palm straight onto the coals for four seconds. Spread out the dough while the grill warms up. Utilize a roller pin to flatten the dough and stop just when it is less than one-fourth inch in thickness on a wide chopping board coated with flour (the form isn't so important). Brus the sides of your dough slightly using olive oil.

4. Place the dough on your grill and let it cook for two to four minutes, or until it has risen and turned slightly brown. Rehash with the other side of the dough.

5. Take the dough out of the grill and arrange it on a side, maintaining a half-inch border around it. Across the dough, distribute some fontina cheese. The chopping board should be strewn about. Distribute the Fraiche across your dough and equally distribute the asparagus and lobster.

   Remove the rind from one half of the lemon and cut thin circles from the other half. Across the tart, distribute the thin-sized lemon wedges. Sprinkle using the olive oil and return to the coldest part of your grill, closing the lid for five to ten minutes to enable the cheese to thaw.

6. Take the tart out of the griddle and set it aside. To taste, season with powdered red pepper, lemon juice, and dill. Cut into slices and eat.

Grilled Honey Lime Shrimp

Yield: 4

Ingredients

- 2 limes or ¼ cup of lime juice, freshly-squeezed
- 2 pounds of deveined, peeled raw shrimp
- ¼ cup of Dijon mustard
- ¼ cup of rice vinegar
- ¼ cup of minced fresh chives

- ½ cup of honey

- 2 teaspoons of salt

- 2 teaspoons of minced fresh garlic

- ½ cup of olive oil, extra-virgin

- 1 teaspoon of pepper

Procedure

1. To prepare the marinade, mix all of the ingredients excluding the shrimp inside a large mixing bowl.

2. Marinate the shrimp for thirty minutes in ½ of the dressing.

3. Using kabob skewers, thread the shrimp onto them.

4. Cook the shrimp for about ten minutes on high heat, turning midway through. Smaller shrimps cook more quickly (approximately five to seven minutes), so modify your cooking time

accordingly. As the shrimps are cooking, baste them with the remainder of the dressing.

Spicy Asian Zucchini with Noodles

Yield: 4-6

Ingredients

Salad

- ¼ cup of cilantro leaves (roughly chopped)
- ½ cup of red cabbage (finely sliced)
- Two big zucchini, cleaned and clipped ends, use a vegetable peeler or spiral cutter to cut into the 'noodles'
- ½ cup of sugar snap peas or snow peas (finely sliced)
- One big carrot, peeled and rinsed, cut into the 'noodles' with a julienne vegetable peeler or spiral cutter

- Two green onions (finely sliced)

Sauce

- Two tablespoons of avocado oil (may be replaced with olive oil)
- One garlic clove (coarsely minced)
- ¼ teaspoon dried ginger (may be replaced with one teaspoon of grated fresh ginger)
- Three tablespoons of coconut aminos
- A pinch of red pepper flakes or cayenne, to taste
- One tablespoon of sesame oil (toasted)
- ½ cup of creamy almond butter (without having added sugar)
- One tablespoon of water
- One lime's juice
- Serve with lime wedges

Procedure

1. Using a handheld vegetable peeler or a spiral vegetable cutter, cut carrots as well as zucchini into

'noodles' or spirals and put in a big mixing bowl (you'll obtain ribbons instead of 'noodles' in this case).

2. Combine green onions, red cabbage, cilantro, as well as snow peas in a large mixing bowl. Set aside after lightly mixing.
3. Whisk combined all the sauce items in a small dish. It will be thick, however after you combine it with the zucchini and 'sweats,' you'll get the correct consistency.
4. Toss the veggies with the sauce and then top with more cilantro. If preferred, garnish using lime wedges.
5. Refrigerate leftovers in an airtight jar for up to two days.

Homemade Salmon Tacos and Salsa

Yield: 4

Ingredients

Tacos:

- Avocado oil (two teaspoons)
- ½ tbsp. of cumin
- ¼ tsp. chili powder
- ½ tsp. of salt
- ½ tsp. of pepper (ground)
- ½ tsp. of garlic powder
- Two corn cobs (brushed with avocado oil and sea salt)
- One sliced avocado
- Four to six tortillas (almond flour made from one gluten-free tortilla)
- One pound of salmon
- ½ pound of purple cabbage (chopped)

Salsa

- Two cloves of garlic

- ½ onion (sweet)
- Two containers of Village Farms True Rebel Mixed tomatoes (Ten oz.)
- ½ de-seeded jalapeno
- A pinch of cilantro
- One lime, freshly squeezed
- 1/4 tsp. of cumin
- ½ tsp. of salt

Procedure

1. Preheat the oven to 662 °C.
2. Arrange the salmon on a baking sheet that has been lined with parchment paper.
3. Drizzle each filet with avocado and season with garlic powder, chili powder, cumin, sea salt, and ground pepper.
4. Sea salt, and ground pepper.
5. Bake for 12-15 minutes in the oven, or until the salmon is no more page and translucent.

6. Break the fish into big slices using a fork. While the fish is in the oven, brush the corn using avocado oil and season with salt and pepper.
7. Preheat the grill on high heat for a few minutes.
8. Put the corn just on the grill as well as cook it for approximately 5 minutes, turning it periodically until it's browned. You may also grill the tortillas to keep them warm but also toast them a little. However, they get brown rapidly, so keep an eye on them!
9. Preparation of salsa: in a food processor, mix all of the salsa ingredients. the procedure for an approximately 5 seconds
10. Scrape down both sides with a rubber spatula then mix again until mixed but yet chunky.
11. Arrange the tacos: Put the corn, salmon, avocado, salsa, and cabbage cut off the Cobb for every tortilla.

12. Squeeze more lime juice over the top and garnish with more cilantro leaves.

Noodle Bowl with Keto Asian Barbecue Meatballs

Yield: 4

Ingredients

Meatballs

- Two tbsp. sesame seed oil
- 1 pound of turkey ground meat or chicken
- One tsp. of fish sauce
- 1/4 cup of minced cilantro
- Two green onions (minced)
- Two garlic cloves (minced)
- One tbsp. of soy tamari
- A half tsp. of salt
- 1/4 cup of minced shiitake mushrooms

- 1/2 tsp. crushed red pepper

Barbecue Sauce

- One tbsp. of rice wine vinegar
- ¼ cup Swerve granulated
- One minced garlic clove
- One tbsp. of sesame seed oil
- Three teaspoons of Sriracha oil
- ¼ cup of tamari
- One tbsp. of freshly grated ginger

Other

- Two packets of shirataki noodles (miracle noodles)
- Eight ounces of Snow peas

Procedure

1. Mix all the meatball items, excluding the oil, inside a large mixing bowl. Make sixteen meatballs out of the mixture.

2. Stir all together with the sauce ingredients in a little bowl and leave aside. Arrange the noodles after preparing them using the package recommendations.

3. In a large 10.5" pan, heat the two tablespoons of sesame oil. When the pan is heated, place each meatball in a single layer. Don't forget to sear each side for two to three minutes till it cooked through then remove and put it away

4. The snow peas are tossed and simmered for one minute, or until they begin to wilt. Re-insert each of the meatballs into the pan then drizzle the sauce on the meatballs and finally cover as well as cook for three minutes on low heat.

5. Remove the lid and continue simmering the sauce till it becomes thick and reduced by half. Serve with miracle noodles on top.

Grilled Chicken Breasts with a Five-Ingredient Lemon Yogurt-Marinated

Yield: 5

Ingredients

- One tsp. of extra virgin olive oil
- ½ cup of Greek yogurt (plain)
- Chicken breasts, 1 ¼ pound (usually 5- small four oz. chicken breasts)
- 1/2 big lemon juice
- 1 ¼ tbsp. of spiced sea salt (Mediterranean) (or make your own)

Procedure

1. Blend the Mediterranean seasoned sea salt, olive oil, yogurt, and lemon juice in a mixing bowl and toss to combine. Stir in the chicken breasts until they are well coated in the marinade. Refrigerate for twenty minutes or up to an hour before serving.

2. Gently oil the grill grate then preheat the grill to moderate range.

3. Remove the chicken from the marinade then lay it on the grill for six to eight minutes on each side, just until the juices content runs clear and also the chicken is no longer pink. Season with salt and black pepper to taste and then remove the extra marinade and toss it out.

4. Serve with potatoes, salad, or whatever you want!

Notes on the Recipe

1. To add zing to the chicken, I want to put two minced garlic cloves and one tsp. of dijon mustard into that same marinade. It's incredible!
2. Mix the following ingredients to make your very own Sea Salt (Mediterranean) for this recipe: ½ tsp. of sea salt, one tsp. of dried oregano, ¼ tsp. garlic powder, ¼ tsp. dried thyme, sprinkle of dried basil, and freshly ground black pepper.

3. To make it taste better than chicken, grilling just few sliced lemons is preferred (which are also tasty)!
4. Moroccan Spices and Eggplant with Tomato Stew

Oat Cakes with Turmeric Salmon

Servings: 4

Ingredients

- 1 salmon can
- ½ cup of oats, old-fashioned
- 1 tablespoon of mustard (dijon)
- ½ teaspoon of lemon rind (grated)
- 2 tablespoons of freshly squeezed lemon juice
- ¼ teaspoon of garlic powder
- 1 teaspoon of turmeric
- 1 teaspoon of black pepper, ground
- 1 gently beaten big egg
- 2 tablespoons of hummus of choice

- 2 cups of arugula

Procedure

1. Using a blender, combine the oats, pulse for about ten seconds, or until everything is finely ground. Place in a mixing basin. In a large mixing bowl, combine the egg, mustard, salmon, and two tablespoons of lemon rind, turmeric, pepper, and salt.
2. Combine ingredients in a mixing bowl.
3. Pour the salmon mixture into a 1/3 cup of the dry measuring cup.
4. In a large frying pan, heat the oil over moderate heat and then pat salmon cakes into the pan as you turn the measuring cup over, the mixture will fall out.
5. Cook for almost two minutes on every side, or till it is golden brown on the bottoms.
6. On a platter, arrange the arugula. Squeezed lemon juice should be drizzled on top. Place the salmon

cakes on top of the arugula. Toss with some hummus and also enjoy!

Notes on the Recipe

Do not however forget to add a pinch of black pepper! Turmeric absorption is increased by the use of black pepper! Whenever you don't have oats on hand, ordinary brown rice flour or gluten-free flour can be used instead.

Sriracha Honey Dressing with Salad of Asian Beef

Servings: 4

Ingredients

- Season with pepper and salt to taste
- 1 teaspoon hot sauce such as Sriracha sauce
- ½ tablespoon of soy sauce (low sodium)
- ¼ cup of canola oil

- 1 head of Bibb lettuce or one bag of watercress
- The juice of a Lime
- Thinly sliced red onion (tiny)
- 1 peeled, pitted, and diced avocado
- 1 pint halved of cherry tomatoes
- 2 teaspoons of honey
- ½ cup of finely sliced English cucumber
- 1 pound of flank steak
- Cilantro leaves (a handful)

Procedure

1. Preheat a cast-iron skillet, grill, or grill pan to moderate temperatures. Sprinkle pepper and salt to the steak to season it and cook it for three to four min per side to moderate. Give it at least five min for the steak to rest before slicing it very thin through the grain.

2. In a mixing bowl, mix the soy sauce, honey, lime juice, and sriracha, along with a little pepper, as the meat rests. Mix in the oil slowly.

3. Flip the steak pieces with the cilantro and veggies in a large mixing basin. Flip the salad with the dressing till it is lightly covered.

Foil Packets with Italian Chicken and Veggies

Yield: 2

Ingredients

- One mid-sized zucchini, 1/4 inch thickly cut
- One mid-sized sliced red bell pepper
- One big tomato, peeled and chopped into large bits
- 2 oz. mushrooms, sliced
- ¼ cup of avocado oil
- ¼ cup of onions, thinly sliced

- 1 tbsp. of fresh rosemary, chopped
- Parmesan cheese, grated for serving (not compulsory)
- 1/2 tsp. of salt
- One tsp. of oregano leaves, dried
- One garlic clove, minced
- One cup of green beans, chopped
- 1/4 tsp. of black pepper
- A pound of skinless, boneless chicken thighs, and cut into one inch pieces

Procedure

1. Preheat the oven to 204 °C. Divide aluminum foil into 4 pieces and also into 12-inch squares each.
2. Mix the green beans, chicken, onions, zucchini, garlic bell pepper, mushrooms, and tomato in a large mixing bowl. Trickle the oil over the oregano, pepper, rosemary, and salt to taste. Flip well to blend.

3. Evenly distribute the mixture among all the foil sheets, putting it down the middle of each sheet. Connect two ends of the foil and then fold them over again to seal it. Firmly fold the sides.

4. Oven the packets for twenty-five minutes, or till the chicken is well cooked, on a rimmed parchment paper.

5. Loosen the top seams of the packets as well as remove them. If using, garnish with Parmesan cheese that is grated. Eat from the plates or eat right out of the packets.

Notes on the Recipe

1. When you seem to have more time, the Dietary regimen provides a terrific selection of slow-cooker cuisine, as well as a full section including how to fill your freezer, pantry, and fridge using keto-friendly essentials.

2. Start giving these Veggie Foil Packets and Italian Chicken a try if you're a seasoned keto pro, a rookie, or just searching for certain low-carb choices. If you enjoy Italian cuisine, you should also try this mozzarella with pesto pasta and zucchini!

Steak Soup with Salsa Verde

Servings: 6 - 8

Ingredients

- One mid-sized peeled and sliced white onion
- One big, peeled and chopped Poblano pepper
- Four cups of vegetable broth (or chicken or beef stock)
- Four garlic cloves, minced and peeled
- Two cups (16 oz.) of store-bought or homemade Salsa Verde
- One pound of steak, chopped into 1/2-inch pieces

- Two tsp. of cumin powder
- To taste with freshly crushed black pepper and sea salt
- One pound of Yukon gold potatoes, sliced into 1/2-inch chunks
- One tbsp. of extra virgin olive oil

Procedure

For the Stovetop

1. In a big stockpot, heat the oil over moderate-high heat. Include the poblano and onion, and cook, turning frequently, for five min, or till the onion becomes translucent and tender. Put in the finely chopped garlic and then sauté for a min more, stirring periodically.
2. Add the rest of the ingredients to a large mixing bowl. Cook till the soup has reached a simmer. Lower the heat to medium-low, close, and simmer

for twenty to thirty minutes, just till the steak is soft.

3. Season to taste using pepper and salt if necessary.

4. Garnish using a variety of your preferred toppings and serve warm. Put it in the fridge for up to three days in a tight container, or place it in a freezer for up to three months.

Pressure Cooker (Instant Pot) Procedure

1. Press the "Sauté" button as well as pour oil into the Pressure Cooker's bowl. When the oil is hot, add the poblano and onion. Cook, stringing periodically, for five to six minutes, just till the onion is translucent and tender.

2. Stir in the finely chopped garlic and then Sauté for a minute more, stirring regularly. Select "Cancel" from the drop-down menu.

3. In the bowl of the Pressure Cooker, mix the rest of the ingredients but also stir gently to blend. Set the lid to "Sealing" and close it tightly. Cook for

twenty min on high pressure, then rapid release. Take off the cover.

4. Season to taste with pepper and salt if necessary.
5. Garnish using a variety of your preferred toppings and serve warm. Store in the refrigerator for up to three days in a tight container, or store in a freezer for up to three months.

Slow Cooker (Crock-Pot) Procedure

1. In the bowl of a big six-quart Crock-Pot, mix all ingredients (except the oil) as well as stir quickly to blend.
2. Close and cook for six to eight hours on low or three to four hours on high, just till the steak is cooked.
3. Season to taste using pepper and salt if necessary.
4. Garnish using a variety of your preferred toppings and serve warm. Store in the refrigerator for up to three days in a tight container, or store in the freezer for up to three months.

Spicy Drunken Noodles

Servings: 3 - 4

Ingredients

- Three minced garlic cloves
- A tablespoon of oyster sauce
- A tablespoon of fish sauce
- Two eggs
- A teaspoon of sugar
- A tablespoon of Sriracha sauce
- Three tablespoons of soy sauce
- Six basil leaves, cut into ribbons and add one cup of loosely packed whole leaves
- Three tablespoons peanut or canola oil
- 1/3 pound of chicken or beef, thinly cut across the grain
- Sliced mid-sized white onion
- 3–4 cups divided rice noodles

- ¼ cup of rice wine
- One or two Serrana peppers, thinly sliced
- 1/2 cup of halved grape tomatoes

Procedure

1. Add the fish sauce, soy sauce, Sriracha, oyster sauce, half of the chopped garlic, sugar, and six Thal basil leaves inside a small mixing bowl.
2. Reserve the mixture when the sugar has dissolved. Heat oil to moderate-high in a big non-stick skillet. Add the remaining garlic and cook for a minute, or till it turns golden, and scramble the eggs for about a minute, or till it is almost set.
3. Put in the onions and meat and simmer for one to two minutes, or till the meat is almost done.
4. Combine the tomatoes, rice noodles, saved sauce, basil leaves, and Serrang peppers in a large mixing bowl. Three to five minutes, stir to incorporate till

the noodles are well cooked and the ends are slightly crunchy. Stir in the rice and wine and serve.

Notes on the Recipe

Whenever you can't get broad, flat noodles, Thai noodles (dried pad) will suffice. Just keep in mind that before you begin cooking, soak them in water using the package instructions.

Banana Berry Breakfast Oat Bars

Servings: 9

Ingredients

For the Base

- ½ cup of out flour
- ¼ teaspoon of Himalayan salt
- 1 ripe banana
- 2 teaspoons of lemon zest, gotten from a lemon

- 1 tablespoon of honey or syrup
- ½ teaspoon of baking powder
- 1 ½ cups of rolled oats
- 1 teaspoon of vanilla extract
- 2 tablespoons of coconut oil (cooled and melted)

For Topping

- One tablespoon of coconut oil (cooled and melted)
- For Raspberry Chia Jam
- One tablespoon of honey or syrup or stevia
- One tablespoon of syrup or honey, to taste and if desired
- One cup of fresh raspberries
- Two tablespoons of chia seeds
- One cup of rolled oats
- One teaspoon of vanilla extract
- ½ cup of fresh blueberries

Procedure

1. Preheat oven to about 190°C and baking sheet an 8"x8" (22cmx22cm) baking pan.
2. Combine the dry ingredients (salt, rolled oats, baking powder, lemon zest, and flour) in a big mixing basin.
3. Smash the banana using a fork in a different basin. Mix in the syrup or honey and vanilla essence until the mixture is smooth.
4. Combine the banana and oat mixture in a mixing bowl. Mix in the coconut oil till it is thoroughly incorporated and dough appears.
5. Place the dough in the baking pan that has been prepared and then the mixture should be pushed down hard and evenly with a spatula or fingers. Leave it for ten min in the oven.
6. Prepare the toppings for the meantime. Combine all ingredients in a mixing bowl. With your hands mix in the coconut oil and stir only till a dough forms.

This shouldn't be crumbly, and it should hold together well. Set aside.

7. Take the pan out of the oven and scatter the raspberry chia jam uniformly over the entire surface. Include blueberries in the mix. Sprinkle the topping mixture gently on top and softly press it down. Make sure to bake for thirty min, or till the top is golden brown.

8. Pull the baking sheet out from the oven and set it aside to cool fully. Enjoy by cutting into bars.

9. To make raspberry chia jam, combine all of the ingredients in a blender and blend until smooth. In a saucepan over low heat, place fresh raspberries. Using a fork, mash the raspberries and then simmer for some minutes, or till the raspberries become soft.

10. Remove from the heat and whisk in the stevia, honey, syrup, or chia seeds. Stir for some minutes, then set aside for 5min while the mixture thickens.

11. Make Banana Berry Breakfast Oat Bars with the jam. Place the remaining jam in a glass jar in the refrigerator. The jam may be stored in the refrigerator for up to one week.

Feta Turkey Burgers with Caramelized Onion Spinach

Servings: 6

Ingredients

- Four tablespoons avocado oil
- One pound of ground turkey
- One cup of packed spinach
- Two pressed garlic cloves
- ½ cup of crumbled feta.
- One chopped onion (sweet)
- ¼ teaspoon of pink Himalayan sea salt
- 1/8 teaspoon of ground pepper

- ¼ teaspoon of cumin
- One washed large sweet potato
- ¼ teaspoon of smoked paprika

Procedure

1. Using a sharp knife, slice the sweet potato into ¼ - ½ inch pieces. Over moderate heat, put them in a big pan with one tbsp. of avocado. Cook for Three min on one side, then turn and cook for yet another two minutes on the other.
2. Cook, flipping occasionally until they are very soft as well as cooked through. Place on a platter with a clean cloth on top and then set aside.
3. Remove the sweet potatoes from the pan and wipe them clean. One tbsp. avocado oil in a skillet with chopped onion over moderate-high heat.
4. Sauté for ten minutes, stirring often, till the onions are browned and reduced. Place the onions in a moderate mixing basin.

5. Include the spinach leaves in the same pan and then sauté for three minutes, or till the spinach is wilted. Place them in the mixing basin. In a mixing basin, combine the smoked paprika cumin, garlic, ground turkey, salt, feta, and ground pepper. Smash it all together with your hands and completely blend it.

6. Warm your pan over moderate-high heat after cleaning it. In the same skillet, include another tbsp. of avocado oil and then form six patties using your hands as well as place them two inches apart in your pan. Cook for three minutes before flipping.

7. Cook for three minutes before flipping. Cook for just a total of ten minutes, or till the sliders are fully cooked.

8. Put the burger between two rounds of sweet potato and top with your favorite toppings.

9. Toppings include sprouts, tomato, lettuce, and avocado to name a few.
10. Serve with your preferred condiments, sit back and enjoy!!

Snapper a la Veracruz

Servings: 4

Ingredients

- 2 tablespoons of capers
- ¼ cup of olive oil
- 1 handful fresh parsley or cilantro, roughly chopped
- ¼ cup of pitted green olives (chopped)
- 1-pint of cherry tomatoes
- Pickled or fresh jalapenos, chopped (not necessary)
- 4 fillets of snapper (or using a firm like cod, halibut, or white fish), four to six ounces each
- Juice of one lime
- Salt to taste

Procedure

1. Preheat the grill to moderate heat. Mix the cherry tomatoes, capers, cilantro or parsley, olives, olive oil, jalapenos, and lime juice, if using, in a mixing basin.
2. 4 sheets of aluminum foil should be folded in half lengthwise, immediately unfolded, and placed on the counter. Sprinkle every fish fillet using salt and arrange it parallel to the fold on one end of the foil. One-fourth of the salsa should be placed at the top of every fillet. Fold the aluminum foil over to completely close the fish, and the next thing is to tightly roll the ends to close the package.
3. Lay the packets just on the grill grate as well as close the lid (the grill temperature should reach roughly 450°F with the lid down). Cook the fillets for eight to ten minutes, or till it is well cooked. Slash the sachets open, just before eating.

Bear-Sized PB and J

Servings: 1

Ingredients

- 1/3 cup of mixed strawberries and blackberries, chopped
- Two freezer waffles, high-protein (like Kodiak)
- Two tablespoons of crunchy peanut butter.
- Two tablespoons of high-protein granola (like Nature Valley)

Procedure

1. Toast your waffles as directed on the packet. Apply the peanut butter on 1 waffle while it's heated.
2. Garnish with granola, berries, and the remaining waffle. Allow cooling completely before covering in aluminum foil. Before you eat, smash. Rolls of spicy tuna in five minutes

Five Mins Spicy Tuna Rolls

Ingredients

- Avocado (cut and slice)
- One cucumber (Cucumber strips should be trimmed and sliced to fit the width of the cucumber strips)
- Salt and Pepper to taste
- 2 teaspoons of Sriracha
- 1 pouch or can of tuna
- 1 tablespoon of mayo (used for mostly tuna mixture)
- 2 teaspoons of garlic powder

Procedure

1. Using a vegetable peeler, cut cucumbers lengthwise into thin strips.
2. Drain tuna when required and combine with pepper, mayo, salt, sriracha, and garlic powder in a

mixing bowl. It is best if the mixture is somewhat moist and not too.

3. Arrange cucumber strips on the work surface and evenly distribute the tuna mixture. Down the strip, keeping about one inch at the ends.
4. Put avocado slices at the end of the cucumber strip above the tuna as well as roll it up firmly.
5. To make the sauce, combine sriracha and mayo and then sprinkle over the cucumber rolls.

Easy and Quick Turkey Noodle Soup

Servings: 6

Ingredients

- ½ chopped medium onion
- Four cups of chicken broth
- Three cloves garlic minced
- Four cups of water
- Two tablespoons of fresh parsley chopped

- Two dashes of Italian seasoning
- Two cups of cooked turkey
- Three medium carrots sliced/chopped
- Three chopped sticks of celery
- Pepper and salt to taste
- Two cups of egg noodles
- Two tablespoons of butter

Procedure

1. In a big soup pot over moderate-high heat, heat the butter to melt. Sauté for five to seven minutes with the celery and onion.
2. Cook for thirty seconds after adding the chopped garlic cloves to the soup pan.
3. In a big soup pan, combine the turkey, water, broth, carrots, and Italian spice.
4. Raise the heat to a higher range and then bring the mixture to a boil.

5. Include the egg noodles in the mixture and lower the heat to maintain a gentle boil. Cook for ten minutes, or till the noodles and carrots are tender. Before dishing, toss in the parsley. Then season with pepper and salt.

Notes on the Recipe

Give the carrots a head start before introducing the egg noodles if you're using bigger carrots or if you don't chop them short.

Cauliflower Enchiladas (Roasted)

Servings: 8

Ingredients

- Toppings lots of chopped fresh cilantro, crumbled queso fresco, sliced avocado, pepitas, etc.
- One batch of basic cauliflower(roasted)
- One batch of red enchilada sauce

- Seven to eight large flour tortillas
- Rinsed as well as drained 2 (15oz.) cans of pinto beans
- 1 (8oz.) bag of shredded cheese (it's to use pepper jack or Mexican blend)

Procedure

1. Preheat the oven to 177 °C. Using cooking spray and lightly butter a 9x13-inch baking pan.
2. Follow the steps for making the red enchilada sauce and roasted cauliflower. When the enchilada sauce is finished, pour ¼ cup of it into the baking pan's bottom and then apply it evenly using a spoon to coat the whole surface. Set Aside.
3. Lay a flattened tortilla on a platter and ladle a generous spoonful of enchilada sauce in the middle. Use a spoon and evenly distribute it. Line down and add ¼ cup of shredded cheese in the center of the

tortilla, followed by a tablespoon of roasted cauliflower and beans.

4. Wrap the enchilada and lay it seam-side down in the prepared pan. Replace the beans, cauliflower, tortillas, and cheese with the remaining beans, cauliflower, tortillas, and cheese. Then put the leftover sauce down the middle of the enchiladas pan as well as distribute it evenly with a spoon.

5. Bake for twenty to twenty-five minutes, exposed, till the tortillas are slightly crunchy and the enchiladas are well cooked.

6. Pull it from the oven, cover it with a variety of toppings, as well as serve immediately.

Sea Salt and Lime Spinach Chips

Yield: 4

Ingredients

- Juice and zest of one large lime (about 2 teaspoons of juice +1 ½ tablespoon of zest), divided
- ½ teaspoon of sea salt
- 8 packed cups of fresh whole spinach leaves, dried and rinsed
- 2 tablespoons of olive oil, extra-virgin

Procedure

1. Have the oven preheated to 275 degrees Fahrenheit. Then, baking sheets should be lightly greased or lined with nonstick pads.
2. Mix the zest and salt inside a small dish with your fingertips.
3. Combine the spinach and the olive oil inside a big mixing basin to coat evenly. Stir in some lime salt and have it tossed one more. to sprinkle a small amount of salt upon every leaf If required, employ your hands.

4. Evenly spread the spinach across the 2 cookie trays that have been prepped. A tsp. of lime juice should be added to each batch.
5. Bake for thirty to thirty-five minutes (contingent on the freshness of your spinach, it may take less time, so pay attention to it) just until the leaflets are shriveled and extremely thin.
6. Take the chips out of the oven and allow them to cool fully on the pan prior to serving.

Four-ingredient Veggies Egg Muffins

Yield: 12

Ingredients

- 15 ½ ounces or 1 can of diced tomatoes plus drained green chilies
- 6 eggs
- ½ cup of shredded Mexican cheese
- ½ cup of milk

Procedure

1. Have the oven preheated to 375°.
2. Combine the milk and eggs in a mixing bowl. Mix in the cheese and chopped tomatoes equally.
3. Spoon the batter into muffin pans (use either slightly lubricated tins or coat the muffin pan using muffin papers).
4. Bake for seventeen to twenty minutes, or until a spoon inserted into the center pulls out clean. Serve right away or keep extras in the fridge for up to 7 days.

Sheet Pan Curried Chicken and Vegetables

Ingredients

- 4 tsp. of Curry powder divided
- 4 tbsp. of divided Olive oil
- 4 cups of Cauliflower florets

- 2 tsp. salt, divided
- 2 Red bell peppers, cut into pieces
- 3 cups of Carrots, cut to form a carrot stick
- 6 bone-in skin-on chicken thighs
- 1 tablespoon shredded fresh ginger
- 1 cup of finely chopped Cilantro
- 2 cups of chopped Green onions

Procedure

1. Have the oven preheated to 450°F.
2. Combine two tsp. of curry powder, one tablespoon of olive oil, and one teaspoon of salt in a large mixing basin. Combine the carrots, cauliflower, ginger, and bell pepper inside the bowl until evenly covered.
3. Put the veggies onto a sheet pan that has been lined or oiled.
4. Combine the remaining two tbsp. olive oil, two tsp. curry powder, and one tsp. salt inside a separate

dish. Stir in the chicken thighs inside the basin until fully lined.

5. Arrange the thighs onto the sheet over the veggies.
6. Take the chicken out of the oven after twenty minutes and garnish the green onions on top of the veggies and chicken. Place the pan in the oven and bake for another ten minutes, or just until the chicken is completely cooked.
7. Take the pan out of the oven and top with cilantro. Have fun!

Very Cherry Protein Shake

Yield: 1

Ingredients

- 1 cup of tart cherry juice
- 1 cup of frozen pitted cherries
- 1 scoop vanilla protein powder
- 1 cup of water

Procedure

1. Combine all of the ingredients inside a blender.
2. Blend until completely smooth. Serve.

Chickpea, Butternut Squash, and Lentil Moroccan Stew

Yield: 4

Ingredients

- 1 medium chopped white or yellow onion
- 1 tablespoon of olive or coconut oil
- 2 tsp. of cumin
- 6 cloves of minced garlic,
- 1 tsp. of ground turmeric
- 1 tsp. of cinnamon
- 28 ounces or 1 can of crushed tomatoes
- ¼ tsp. of cayenne pepper
- 15 ounces or 1 can of chickpeas, drained and rinsed

- 2 ½ cup of organic low sodium vegetable broth
- 1 cup of thoroughly rinsed green lentils
- 4 cups of cubed butternut squash (from about two lb. butternut squash)
- Black pepper, freshly ground
- ½ tsp. of salt
- 1/3 cup of cilantro, chopped
- Fresh juice of half a lemon
- **Optional**: a few leaves of chopped basil

Procedure

1. Inside a big pot, heat the oil on moderate-high heat. Cook for some minutes, or to the point where the onion softens, before adding the garlic and onion.
2. Add the cinnamon, cumin, cayenne, and turmeric and simmer for thirty seconds to one minute, until aromatic.

3. Combine the broth, tomatoes, butternut squash, chickpeas, pepper, salt, and lentils in a large mixing bowl. Allow to boil, then lower to a gentle heat and cook for approximately twenty minutes, or until there is a softening of the butternut squash and the lentils in the pot are thoroughly cooked.

4. Add the juice and, if preferred, the basil and cilantro. If you're not vegan, top with a spoonful of yogurt.

Low-carb Turkey Cabbage Rolls

Yield: 6

Ingredients

- 2 teaspoons of olive oil
- 1 large green cabbage
- 1 minced medium yellow onion
- 1 pound of lean ground turkey

- 2 celery stalks, chopped into half-inch pieces
- 3 cloves of minced garlic
- 1 tablespoon of dried oregano
- ¾ cup of baby carrots, chopped into half-inch pieces
- 2 teaspoons of dried thyme
- 2 teaspoons of dried basil
- Pepper and Salt to taste
- 52 ounces or 1 large bottle of crushed tomatoes

Procedure

1. Preheat the oven to 375 degrees Fahrenheit. Make a square shape in the bottommost part of the cabbage, then an X shape in the middle. Remove the core and throw it away.

2. Fill a big saucepan halfway with water and let it boil. Close and submerge the cabbage with the core side facing the water. boil for six minutes.

3. Preheat a big pan over medium-high heat as the cabbage is still boiling. Allow the turkey to brown before adding it to the pan. Move the turkey towards the sides and stir in the garlic and onions until they begin to brown. Combine the herbs, carrots, and celery in a large mixing bowl. After three minutes, put 1/2 of the smashed tomatoes, a bit of pepper, and a bit of salt.

4. So when cabbage is finished boiling, transfer it to a strainer inside the sink to chill. Remove the outer leaves with tongs and set them on a platter. Put the cabbage into the heated water for yet another two minutes after you see the remaining interior leaves are still somewhat raw. Return the leaves to the colander and let them cool before adding them to your dish.

5. Spread a thin layer of smashed tomatoes on the bottommost part of a ceramic or glass baking dish. Cut the tough stem out of a cabbage leaf and place

it on a big dish. 3/4 cup of filling should be placed in the center of the leaf. Fold in three sides, then wrap it up like a burrito, burying the end beneath. Fill the baking sheet halfway with water. Carry on with the rest of the filling and leaves.

6. Pour the remaining smashed tomatoes on the cabbage rolls after the casserole dish is filled. Bake for thirty minutes, unclosed. Allow to cool before serving.

Oven-roasted Butternut Squash

Yields: 4

Ingredients

- 1 tbsp. of chopped rosemary
- 2 pounds or 1 butternut squash, peeled, seeded, chopped into one-inch cubes
- 2-3 tbsp. of olive oil
- 1 tbsp. of chopped thyme leaves

- 2 cloves of minced garlic
- Squeeze lemon
- Pepper and salt to taste

Procedure

1. Preheat the oven to 400 degrees Fahrenheit. Spray a baking sheet with Pam or vegetable spray and line it with tin foil or parchment paper.
2. Combine the thyme, rosemary, squash, pepper, and salt in a large mixing dish. Toss the squash in the oil to coat it.
3. Arrange in one layer on the lined baking sheet.
4. Cook for twenty minutes. Rearrange squash in a single layer after stirring. Do   minutes roasting time
5. Take the squash out of the oven. Stir in the chopped garlic to coat the squash. Shake the veggies out into a layer and roast for another five

minutes, or until the garlic is aromatic but not brown.

6. Take out of the oven and stir with 1/2 a lemon juice. Serve.

Strawberry Avocado Farro Salad

Yields: 4

Ingredients

- 2 ½ cups of vegetable stock or water
- 1 cup uncooked farro
- 1 diced ripe avocado
- ½ pound of California Strawberries, sliced and hulled
- 2 ounces of crumbled goat cheese
- ½ cup of fresh basil leaves
- 2 tablespoons of olive oil
- 2 tablespoons of red wine vinegar or blush wine vinegar

- A pinch of sea salt
- ½ tablespoon of honey
- Pinch freshly cracked black pepper

Procedure

1. Bring stock or water to a boil inside a mid-sized pot. Cook for twenty-five to thirty minutes, covered, with farro.
2. Turn off the heat and let it drain any leftover liquid. Allow the farro to cool fully before serving.
3. Toss chilled farro with chopped avocado, sliced California strawberries, crumbled goat cheese, and basil leaves in a large mixing dish.
4. Combine the other ingredients into a small mixing dish. Pour the dressing over the farro salad. Toss gently to cover. Serve immediately or keep refrigerated until you are prepared to use.

Golden Milk Chia Pudding

Yield: 1

Ingredients

- 3 tablespoons of chia seeds
- 1 cup of milk
- 1/8 teaspoon of black pepper
- 1 teaspoon of turmeric powder
- Pinch of cardamom and cinnamon
- 1 tablespoon of honey
- 1 small knob of fresh ginger

Procedure

1. Simmer the milk with turmeric, 1 tablespoon cardamom, black pepper, honey, ginger, and cinnamon inside a small saucepan. Take out of the heat and set aside to cool. Using a strainer, take the ginger out of the milk.

2. Pour the milk into a jar or a container. Stir in the chia seeds and the milk.

3. Close the container/jar and place it in your refrigerator all night.

4. Check for sweetness and add additional honey if necessary. If desired, garnish with fruits and nuts just before you serve.

Perfect Steak Fajitas

Yield: 4

Ingredients

For the meat preparation

- Pepper and salt to taste
- 2 tbsp. of taco seasoning
- 1 lime
- 2 large flank steaks.
- Olive oil

For the preparation of the vegetable

- 1 yellow pepper
- 1 green pepper
- 2 large red onions
- 1 yellow pepper
- 1 lime (or more depending on their juiciness/size)
- 1 large yellow onion
- 8 warmed small flour tortillas

For the sliced avocado

- Cilantro
- Sour cream
- Salsa (homemade or jarred)

Procedure

1. In a large mixing bowl, combine the pepper, salt, taco seasoning, lime juice, and a generous drizzle of olive oil. Incorporate the steaks and make sure

they are completely coated inside the marinade. Reserve it somewhere safe.

2. Remove the seeds and cut the peppers to form thin strips. Cut the onions into thin slices after peeling them. Prepare any additional garnishes to go with the fajitas. To rest the steak, get some aluminum foil and a plate prepared.

3. Sear the steak: Inside a stainless steel pan over moderate-high heat, have the meat heated. Take the meat out of the marinade and set aside any leftovers. Sear the meats on each side for two to three minutes, or until it becomes browned and effortlessly removed from the pan. Don't overcook the food. Place the ready plate on top of the pan and close securely with aluminum foil. Reserve somewhere safe.

4. Cook the veggies: Return the pan to a moderate-high heat setting and incorporate any remaining marinade. Have the veggies stir-fried for about four

to five minutes, or until they are soft. If they char a bit, that's alright. Turn the heat up to high and allow the pan to sizzle. Remove the pan from the heat after adding the lime juice to it and tossing

5. Using a sharp knife, gently cut the meat to form strips. Warm wheat tortillas and your desired toppings will go well with the veggies and meat.

Made in the USA
Middletown, DE
16 April 2023